Mommy has a Boo-Boo

Explaining Breast Cancer To Children

Written By
Marci Greenberg Cox

Illustrated By Brooke Foster

Mommy has a Boo-Boo

Library of Congress Control Number: 2021919301
ISBN: 978-1-7367038-3-0
Printed in the United States of America

www.florpublishing.com

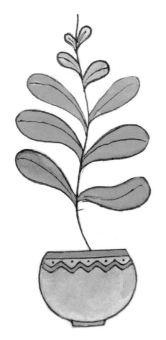

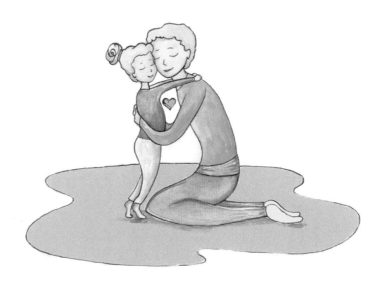

Dedicated to my daughters:
Jewelz, Lily, and Autumn
May you find strength within you.

Mommy has a boo-boo in her boobies that made her sick.

You can't see the boo-boo. It's different than the kind of boo-boo you get if you fall off your bike and scrape your knee—or if you trip at the park and need a bandage.

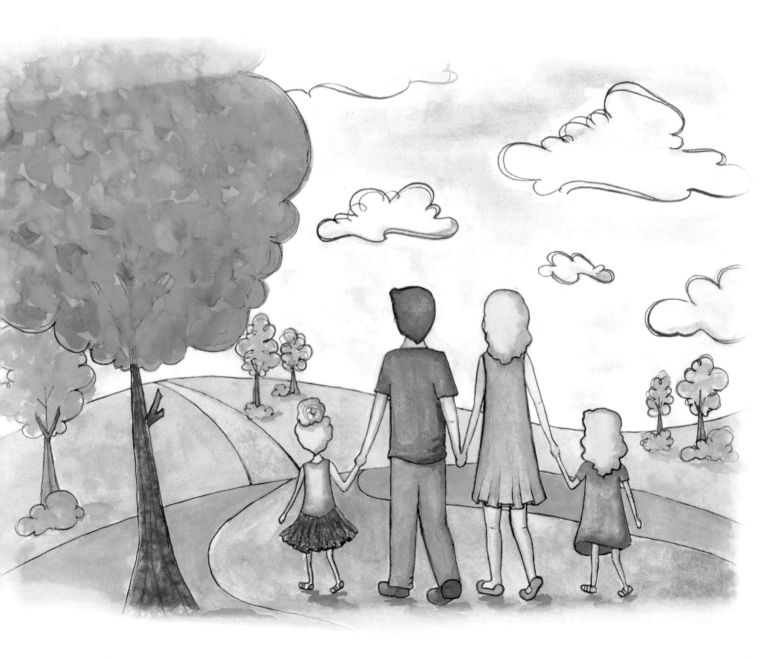

Mommy needs to get the boo-boo fixed, but first she has to meet with doctors so they can make a plan.

The doctors call Mommy's boo-boo cancer.

What does that mean?...

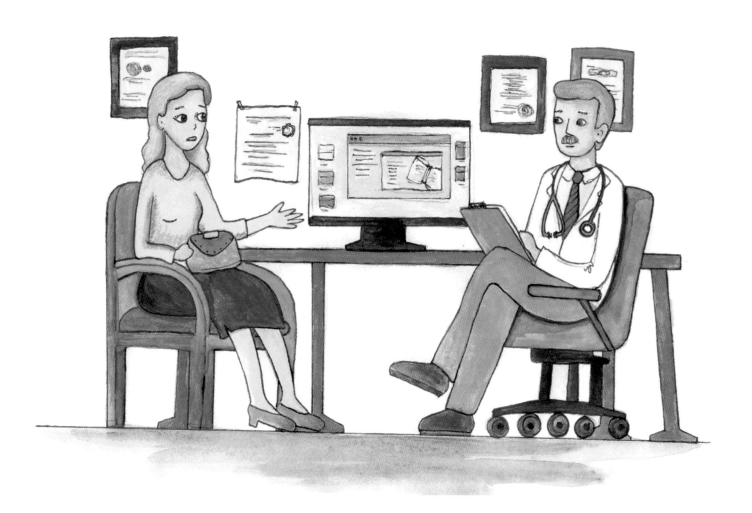

Cancer is not a cold that you catch.

But cancer can make a body feel sick.

Cancer can cause a lump or bump in the body that is not supposed to be there.

Mommy is going to take medicine and have treatments to make that boo-boo lump called cancer go away. Mommy might even lose her hair, but the doctors are helping her get better soon!

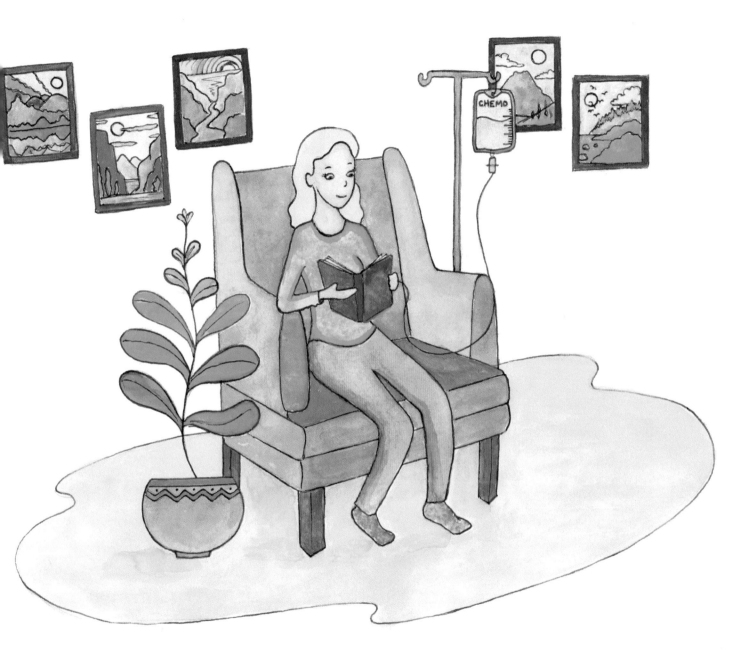

Mommy is having surgery to get the cancer out of her body.

No more boo-boo!

The surgery won't hurt Mommy because the doctors give her medicine that helps.

Mommy is going to feel better!

You are not sure about surgery, but Mommy is safe. She is in good hands.

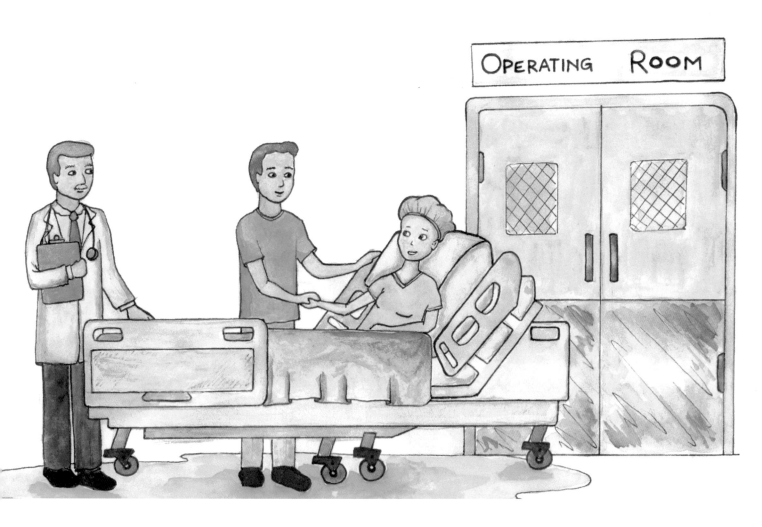

The surgery is over, and Mommy's boo-boo is gone.

And.... Her boobies are gone, too. Mommy is very happy about this!

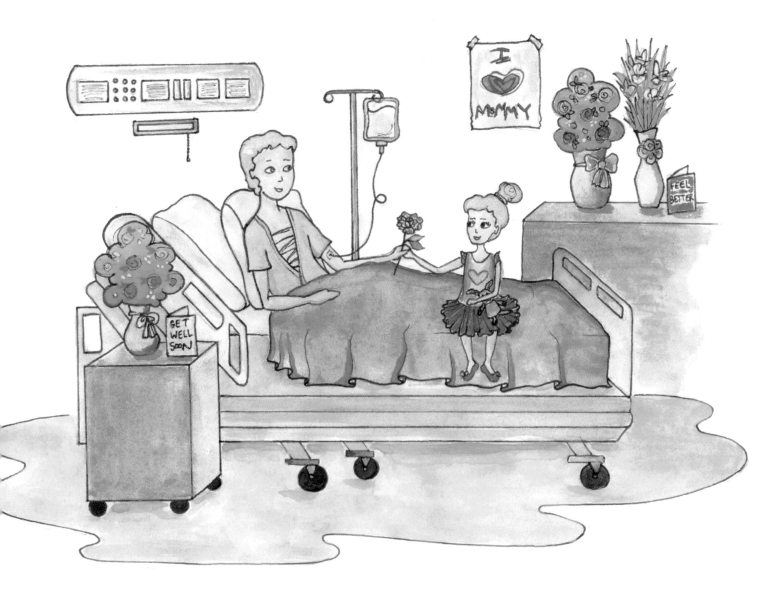

Mommy gives you a great, big hug and kiss!

You can feel all of her love.

With no more boobies, when Mommy gives you a great big hug you are even closer to her heart!

(Can you feel it beating a song of love for you?)

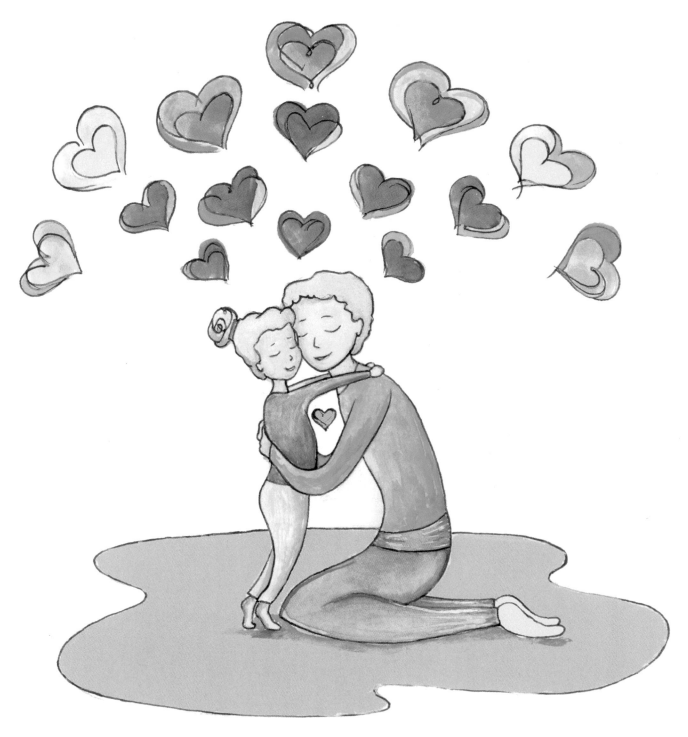

You are a great help to Mommy while she is healing from surgery. She needs to take it easy, she explains. Cancer takes time to heal and she still has to see doctors and be on medication.

Mommy feels tired and she might need to take a break from playing. She has a happy feeling watching you and your sister have fun together! She says thank you for helping clean up the toys. Thank you for getting her a blanket so she can take a little nap. (Do you want to take a nap, too?)

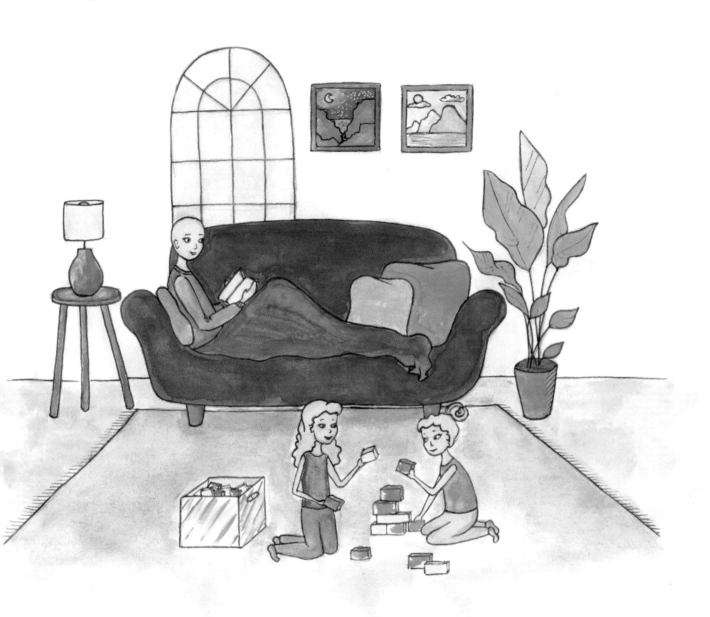

After some time, Mommy is feeling much better. She is not ready to lift you up super-high or have a dance party just yet!

But soon...

She is always ready to hold you close to her heart and give you a big hug and kiss!

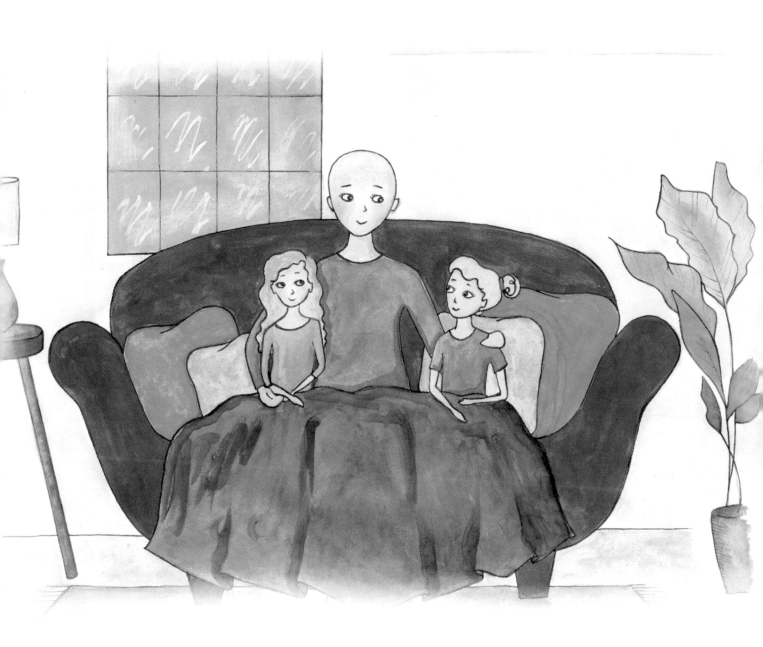

Mommy looks different because her boobies are gone.

Her boo-boo is gone, too. Mommy is getting better!

Mommy looks different, but SHE is the same!

Mommy loves you!

Mommy Had a Boo-Boo but now it's gone!

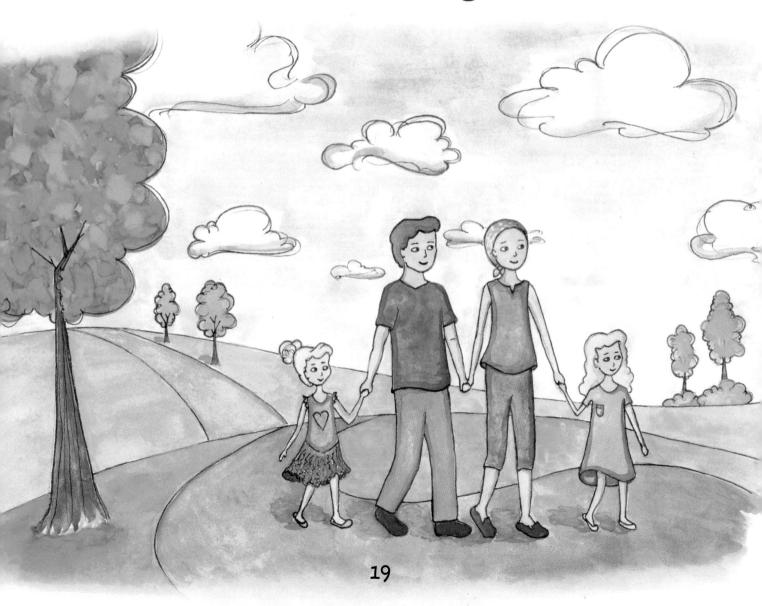

About the author:

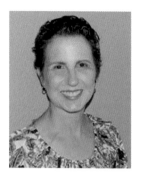

Marci Greenberg Cox is a first time author. After being diagnosed with Stage 3 invasive ductal carcinoma in November 2018 she decided to not have reconstruction. She wanted to write a book to help other mom's explain to their children about not having breasts anymore. Marci lives in Glendale, AZ, where she enjoys spending time with her husband and daughters, crafting and working as a full time REALTOR.

About the illustrator:

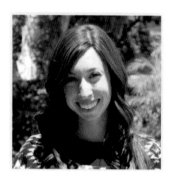

Brooke Foster is an artist, teacher, and mama living in Phoenix, Arizona with her husband and two daughters. She grew up with a passion for drawing and moved to Arizona to attend Arizona State University, where she graduated with a BFA in Fine Arts. She is always creating, whether it is a commissioned project or just a fun art activity with her little ones. Her favorite materials are watercolor and ink, which she used to create the illustrations for this book!

About the editor:

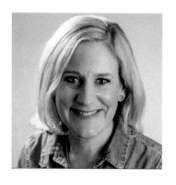

Kristen Hampshire is a freelance journalist who has contributed to U.S. News, HGTVRemodels.com and a range of consumer and trade magazines focused on home, business, health and education. She regularly writes for Cleveland magazine and a host of custom publications. She is a book collaborator and author of a series of home and garden books published by Quayside. Kristen started WriteHand Co. in 2004 after serving as an editor for several years. She has been recognized as "Best In Ohio: Freelancer" by the Press Club of Cleveland, and a Young Scholar by the American Society of Business Press Editors (ASBPE). Kristen lives in Bay Village, Ohio, where she enjoys time with her two children, kayaking on the Lake Erie, running and knitting.

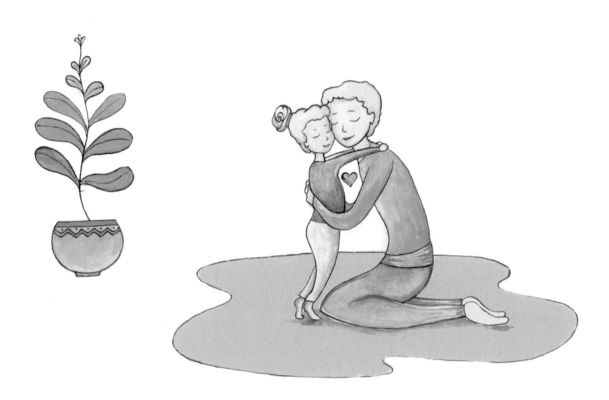

Illustrated by Brooke Foster
Edited by Kristen Hampshire

Made in the USA
Middletown, DE
30 March 2022